Superfoods

Top 20 Superfoods You Should be Eating

By
Bring on Fitness

About Bring On Fitness

Our passion for fitness gave life to **Bring On Fitness**. We started with the goal of helping as many people as we can. To educate, motivate and to help change peoples lives for the better. Bring On Fitness is not only for the fitness enthusiasts, but also for the beginner. We strongly believe nothing is more important than learning the basics and creating a strong foundation in both nutrition - through meal planning, and in exercise - by following a specific plan. This is just as important for the beginner, as it is for the experienced athlete.

We set high standards for ourselves, the information we share, and the products we carry. Our goal is to provide you with exceptional products that suit your needs and the knowledge and motivation to help you work towards and achieve your health and fitness goals.

Check us out at www.bringonfitness.com

"Our Mission is to have a positive impact in changing peoples lives. We will deliver the best possible fitness and nutrition solutions that will empower people to achieve their health and fitness goals."

Table of Contents

Introduction

I want to thank you for choosing this book, *"Superfoods: Top 20 Superfoods You Should be Eating."*

Unlike superheroes, superfoods don't come with a cape on, which makes it difficult for us to identify them. Honestly, the term "superfood" is being thrown around so loosely in the media that it leaves us completely overwhelmed, but seriously, how do you define superfood? What exactly is it? Do we need to load up on these so-called superfoods to lead a healthy life? The answer is a definite "yes." Yes, we need superfoods to enhance our lives and protect us from potential health problems.

When I first started noticing signs of lethargy, I passed it off as a symptom of stress, but when the signs persisted, I was forced to take a close look at my dietary habits. Then it dawned on me that my meals were low in nutrition, vitamins, protein, and fiber. We are all guilty of conveniently blaming our lack of nutrition on our busy lifestyles, but we all know that's not the story. Our ignorance is costing us our health, and it's about time we took control of our nutritional needs.

We wanted our readers to have a perfect list of superfoods, which will help them to make healthier choices and, as a result, lead a healthier lifestyle. If you are looking to improve your health or wanting to lose weight, this book presents you with detailed information on 20 superfoods that can change your life. The benefits of each of these superfoods have been carefully studied. The book explains how these superfoods can enhance your overall health.

I sincerely hope that this book ends your search for the best superfoods in the market. Happy reading!

Superfood 1: Broccoli

Who loves broccoli? Okay, I don't know many who would be excited at the thought of eating broccoli. It is a constant struggle to get your kids to eat it and, in some cases, even adults battle to eat broccoli. However, I can assure you that many people who claim to not like broccoli don't know how to cook it the right way.

Broccoli doesn't always have to taste bland. You can always sauté it with spices, soy sauce, or even make smoothies out of it. You can also add it to your salads, add it to several dips, or even bake it by seasoning it with some salt and pepper.

Broccoli is like the underdog of super foods. It may not get as much credit as it deserves, but it's packed with nutrients that can fight cancer. It's loaded with protein, calcium, vitamin C, Vitamin B6, lots of fiber, and magnesium. It also contains a lot of antioxidants, which can fight against aging.

If your goal is to lose weight, there's nothing more satiating and nutrient-rich than broccoli without adding many calories to your diet. If that isn't enough, it also helps in keeping you from developing any heart disease, and it fights congestion. Seriously, there's so much more to these "mini trees" than you know. So the next time you make a trip to the grocery store, don't forget to pick a head of broccoli.

Superfood 2: Avocado

Avocados are everywhere. Avocados seem to have gained a lot of popularity in the past few years because of their nutrient-dense properties. This super-green fruit is the darling of the produce section. They are the absolute go-to ingredient for a guacamole dip. So what makes this pear-like fruit such a hit among people? They are easy to love owing to their flavor, freshness, and the versatility they add to the menu. Regardless of whether you are a health conscious person or not, you will end up falling in love with this fruit.

Avocados contain protein, fiber, vitamin E, potassium, and antioxidants and are low in pesticides. They are known to help you fight sugar cravings and hunger. They lower stress, add satiety to meals, and also cause a reduction in the inflammation of the arteries and the digestive tract. Additionally, avocados often benefit people with type 2 diabetes and those suffering from heart issues.

You want to choose the best avocados when you are out shopping, so we advise that you pick the ripest ones that can be easily digested. To test out an avocado, try peeling off the tiny brown stone at the end. If it's slightly green, consider it healthy, but if it appears brown, it's certainly past its prime, and you need to pick another.

Superfood 3: Sweet Potatoes

Can you guess what most people struggle with when it comes to following a specific diet or eating healthy? They have to give up on sweets, and it can be extremely difficult, especially if you have a sweet tooth like me, but have you considered including creamy textured sweet potatoes to your meals? It's about time you did. You may be surprised to know how versatile they are. These babies can be used for making desserts, starters, curries, and even soups.

Moreover, they are cheap, so if you are a little tight on your pocket, you can still pig out on these "yams" as they are referred to in America. Now there are two types of sweet potatoes: the pale and creamy ones and the ones with bright orange flesh. You can pick whichever you like based on the texture.

These tubers are considered to be extremely rich in vitamins A, C, and B6, as well as fiber, and they are a great source of carbohydrates. The orange-fleshed sweet potatoes are also packed with beta-carotene. Traditionally, sweet potatoes are baked, mashed, or even roasted. However, these days, people are adding them to almost every dish you can think of. Risotto, pasta, noodles and curries – you name it.

Sweet potatoes also contain manganese and some antioxidants that have anti-cancer properties. They also have a low glycemic index as compared to white potatoes and therefore make a better pre-workout meal to give you that extra push needed for an intense workout session. If you are big on strength training, you should include sweet potatoes in your diet.

Superfood 4: Kale

We have been hearing a lot about kale these days. It's so overwhelming that you want to pass it off as one of those health fads that die down with the trend, but no, this veggie needs some serious attention. There's a reason why kale is deemed as the king of the greens. If you didn't know this already, it's considered to be one of the most nutrient-dense veggies across the globe. Yes, across the globe. So if you have been ignoring these super green leaves that are typically lying in the periphery of the store, give them a go.

From helping people to alleviate pain to enhancing heart health or even protecting people from cancer, kale can indeed be called a superfood. One cup of kale consists of different minerals, such as potassium and magnesium, and vitamins A, C, K, and B6. It also provides omega-3 fatty acids. Now that's what I call packing a punch!

Kale isn't as boring as you think. You can use it in different salads or smoothies, and it can even be baked as chips. This vibrant looking veggie, if eaten on a regular basis, can help lower cholesterol, fight against cancer, and also help you shed those excess pounds. Eating kale is also a good way of boosting your iron levels after your workouts.

Superfood 5: Spinach

I know you have heard enough about spinach over the years. By now, whenever you hear about the goodness of spinach, some of you may yawn, but do you know how important this original super green is? Okay, before I talk about its health benefits, let's talk a little about how it can make our meals tastier.

If you have had a long day at work, you can simply make a spinach soup with some tomatoes in it. Season it with some salt and pepper, and you have a refreshingly tasty soup, which will not only soothe your taste buds but will also leave you feeling satiated. Spinach can also be used to make various types of curries, be added to a salad, rice, noodles, pasta, and wraps, and can even be sautéed. Moreover, spinach smoothie could make an excellent breakfast drink after your workout sessions.

As far as its health benefits are concerned, spinach is loaded with calcium, iron, potassium, zinc, vitamin A, beta-carotene, and manganese, among a few others. The nutrients present in spinach can be excellent for your brain function, eyes, and blood pressure levels and can boost your metabolism. Spinach also contains a lot of water-soluble vitamins, minerals, fat-soluble vitamins, and several phytonutrients. According to a particular study, a bowl of spinach is enough to increase your muscle efficiency and to fight against inflamed muscles. This list can go on and on. The bottom line is that you should not forget to include this superfood in your daily diet.

Superfood 6: Green Tea

Almost everyone is seen sipping on some green tea these days. A few months ago, every other person I would bump into would go on and on about how green tea has helped him or her lose weight.

To be honest, I thought this ingredient is too hyped up, so I didn't want to try it. However, here's what happened. I suddenly decided to give it a go, and it did wonders for my health and skin. I believe what they say about green tea – that it's the healthiest drink on this planet. Although green tea is mostly famous among fitness-conscious people, everyone who needs a quick boost of refreshing energy before they start their day can enjoy it.

Aside from boosting your metabolism and helping you lose a few pounds, green tea also offers a plethora of other benefits. These may include:

- Reduced blood pressure levels
- Improved bone density
- Improved memory
- Prevention of cancer
- Reduced risk of heart disease and arteriosclerosis
- Reduced cholesterol levels

Green tea is rich in antioxidant; it helps you detox your skin and leaves it radiant, which will not go unnoticed. If you still have some lingering questions in your mind about green tea, such as "Does it work for everyone?" "Does it have too much caffeine?" or "How much is too much?" let me tell you that your concerns are imaginary. Absolutely anyone, regardless of age or health condition, can gulp down two to three cups of green tea per day without causing any problems.

Superfood 7: Apples

Do I need to say anything more about the goodness of apples? Eating an apple a day to keep the doctor away might be such a clichéd statement that sometimes, you may take this fruit for granted. However, let's accept it. The reputation this fruit has gained over the years is well-deserved.

Apples are one of the healthiest snacks you can have any time of the day without worrying about adding calories. This classic fruit is known to keep a host of illnesses away. This may include obesity, cancer, cholesterol, and the risk of stroke, and it increases brain power. Apples contain enough fiber to keep constipation at bay. They also keep you feeling full for a long time without adding many calories.

So if you are trying to lose weight, apples are your go-to snack. Apples contain antioxidants, flavonoids, vitamins B and C, and a lot of dietary fiber.

Superfood 8: Flaxseeds

Flaxseeds are slowly gaining popularity as the new wonder food on the market. Today, flaxseeds are found in almost all foods, including waffles, crackers, and even oatmeal. Along with consumer demand, the agricultural demand for flaxseeds is rising. These nutty, shiny seeds have a lovely earthy aroma. They are filled to the brim with natural goodness and are extremely versatile.

Some nutrition experts suggest that it's better to consume flaxseeds in ground form to reap the maximum benefits. Finding creative techniques to add flaxseeds to your meals isn't a challenge anymore. People are adding them to practically every dish you can think of: cookies, muffins, bread, smoothies, and desserts – you name it.

Despite it being popular, not many people know about the benefits of flaxseeds. One tablespoon of flaxseeds contains about 40 calories that include 2.8 g of carbohydrates, 2.8 g of fats, 1.6 g of protein, up to 8 g of fiber, and 3 mg sodium. The health benefits of regular consumption of flaxseeds are numerous. Some of these include cancer prevention, regulation of bowel functions, and reduced risk of heart disease.

Superfood 9: Beetroot

Haven't we always known that beetroot is good for us? So why is it that we ignore this wonderfully nutritious vegetable? Do you know what would happen if we all consumed beetroot almost every day? Here's your answer: you would have better stamina, better mood, lower blood pressure, and better blood circulation.

If you haven't yet included this veggie in your meals, it's about time you did. Beetroot is packed with betaine, which can help you against chronic diseases and can protect your internal organs. Traditionally, beetroot was used to cure a wide range of ailments, including skin problems, fever, and constipation. It is also a great source of folate, iron, betaine, magnesium, nitrates, and other antioxidants.

One of the most common ways of consuming beetroot is by juicing it. However, if you are not a juice person, you can add it to salads, rice, noodles, and even desserts. Consuming a medium-sized beetroot before your workouts can instantly boost your performance. It also helps in muscle recovery and prevents hunger. Powdered beetroot is easily available in the market. So if you are missing a bit of sweetness in your meals, you can add a spoonful to your porridge bowl, oats, or even breakfast smoothies. Another way of adding beetroot to your diet is to use the new Beetroot Sprinkle. This super sprinkle from Primrose's Kitchen can be added to smoothies, protein shakes, and even pancakes.

Superfood 10: Goji Berries

Some varieties of Goji berries are overwhelmingly bitter, and that is probably the only reason you have been avoiding this magical super food. However, the dried Goji berries are a bit more palatable with a slightly bitter taste, a sweet aftertaste, and more tartness.

I was also hesitant to try them out because my friends would keep talking about their bitter taste. It's not like I ended up loving them at the first go, but these exotic-looking berries grew on me. You can certainly develop a taste for Goji berries as you keep eating them. This super food can be found in dried form, too, but you may struggle to find the fresh berries.

Goji berries aren't new to the market. In fact, they have been used for centuries in ancient Chinese medicine. In Chinese medicine, these berries are added to blood and immune tonics as they are full of vitamin C, which instantly boosts your immune system. They are also packed with iron and vitamin A, and they consist of an entire set of eight essential amino acids. One ounce of Goji berries contains 3 g of fiber and 4 g of protein.

Moreover, they are low in calories, contain 0% fat, loaded with beta-carotene, and excellent for the eyes and skin. A handful of Goji berries have the power to nourish your kidneys and liver, thus normalizing blood flow and promoting cardiovascular health. A 45-minute workout session calls for at least two tablespoons of Goji berries, as they can help you restore lost electrolytes and enable your muscles to recover quickly.

Superfood 11: Garlic

There are so many reasons to love garlic. This small but humble-looking veggie can turn an ordinary dish into a flavorful treat. It's hard to imagine an Asian, French, or Italian kitchen without this ingredient. However, its ability to bring flavors to a dish is not the only thing that is great about garlic. It plays a significant role in promoting your health, too. This flavor-enhancer has been found effective in fighting cancer, promotes cardiovascular health, has anti-viral and inflammatory properties, and can cure a variety of other ailments, such as cerebral aging, immune disorders, cataracts, arthritis, and even arteriosclerosis.

When you cut or crush garlic, it produces Allicin, which is responsible for the odor as well as the super biological activity of garlic. A clove of garlic offers a variety of compounds, including potassium, zinc, arginine, phosphorus, selenium, and polyphenols. Additionally, it also contains vitamin C, vitamin B6, and some highly effective antioxidants that can slow down your aging. Garlic extract can be used to treat yeast infections and offers protection against prostate enlargement. You can use this ingredient to bring flavors to soups, rice, noodles, pasta, pizza, sizzlers, and even snacks. Burnt garlic soup is considered to be excellent for boosting your immunity, not to mention its irresistible taste.

Superfood 12: Coconut

Did you notice that coconut is having a bit of a moment? There is a huge band of growing supporters – which includes scientists – who are all praises for the healing and restorative properties of coconut. Now there's a lot of debate over whether coconut should be classified as super food, but honestly, there are too many reasons for us not to consider it as one. Coconut can be a lifesaver!

Not a lot of people realize that coconut is immensely effective in stabilizing cholesterol, blood sugar levels, hydration, healing, and can even replace blood plasma in case of emergencies. In ancient India, coconut palm was considered an immune booster, antiviral, antibiotic, antibacterial, and antifungal remedy for centuries. Owing to its high antioxidant characteristics, coconut can be used to:

- Improve digestion
- Lower cholesterol
- Fight viruses
- Ward off wrinkles
- Lose weight
- Regulate hormones
- Fight infections
- Kill bacteria
- Prevent memory loss
- Stabilize glucose levels
- Improve digestion
- Enhance metabolism

Here are a couple more reasons why you should eat coconut.

Coconut water:

Coconut water is not only an extremely soothing drink, but it also contains the highest concentration of electrolytes found in nature. The hard shell of the coconut keeps the water sterile and this makes it perfect for blood transfusions. You can also use it for preparing milkshakes, juices, and soups.

Coconut oil:

Edible coconut oil can be used for baking as well as cooking. Organic coconut oil can help your skin get rid of acne and dangerous toxins. It lends your skin a perfect mix of antioxidants and hydration that keeps it looking younger and smoother. It can also work wonders for your hair by giving it the much-needed nourishment.

Superfood 13: Hemp Seeds

Hemp seeds look like tiny sunflower seeds, have a nutty flavor, a soft texture, and are loaded with nutrients. Hemp seeds are a true gift of Mother Nature. Now, you must have heard a lot about hemp seeds, but you are still unsure about adding it to your meals owing to some random drug tests at your office.

While it's natural for anyone to feel worried as hemp seeds resemble marijuana, they are a completely different branch of cannabis and consists of a very tiny amount of delta-9-tetrahydrocannabinol or THC, which is why marijuana is popular. Hemp seeds can be added to sandwiches, burgers, patties, soups, pasta, muffins, shakes and even granola.

Hemps seeds can offer a pretty large dose of omega-6 and omega-3 fatty acids and also contain anti-inflammatory properties. Hemp seeds make a perfect ingredient for your daily diet if you have arthritis, asthma, multiple sclerosis, psoriasis, eczema, hay fever, and even seasonal allergies.

Aside from holding an abundance of nutrition, three tablespoons of hemp seeds contain as high as 11 g of protein. It's also easy to digest so that you can bid goodbye to constipation, inflammation, and super mortifying flatulence. These seeds are also rich in iron, zinc, and magnesium. Still need a reason to add them to your diet? Don't overthink, and start including them in your meals right away.

Superfood 14: Wheatgrass

While wheatgrass is considered a healthier food option for our four-legged friends, not many are aware how beneficial it can to be humans as well. This baby wheat plant is sprouted, contains high energy, lots of nutrients, as well as live enzymes. Wheatgrass is packed with all the nine essential amino acids, vitamins, chlorophyll, and minerals.

Drinking wheatgrass juice is known to enhance digestion, prevent the bad bacteria from affecting the digestive tract, and reduce cholesterol. It can also give positive results to people suffering from diabetes, anemia, cancer, and certain skin conditions. The best part about wheatgrass is that it's readily available in almost all cafes where they offer shots of wheatgrass. This drink oxidizes your body within no time and extracts the maximum nutrients.

If you are not quite up for gulping down a cup of grassy goodness yet, don't fret; we have something for you, too. Wheatgrass is now available in pill form, too. You can add it to a range of drinks, salads, and smoothies. Its powdered form can be bought from any organic grocery store and can be easily sprinkled on various dishes. If you ever feel the sluggish, can't-get-out-of-that-bed syndrome, consider drinking a shot of wheatgrass. You will instantly feel a boost of energy that will get you going. Drinking a glass of wheatgrass juice is also an excellent way of passing oxygen into your bloodstream, making it a perfect post-workout drink.

Superfood 15: Almonds

When hunger strikes, it can be difficult to stay away from sweet or greasy foods, but neither of them does any good to your waistline. Instead, why not snack on some toasted almonds? It's a much healthier and tastier option than those fried munchies. Almonds are by far the most diet-friendly nuts as they contain enough protein and are extremely heart friendly, owing to increased levels of MUFAs. They also pack enough calcium and fiber as compared to other nuts and are a good source of vitamin E. Given their versatility, almonds can be added to almost all dishes, shakes, and smoothies.

When added to cakes, almonds can bring a highly tasty nutty flavor and an aroma to die for. This superfood boasts a myriad of health benefits, from keeping you safe from chronic diseases to boosting your immune system and even managing menopausal symptoms.

Do you know that almonds can help you fight your weight problems? Almonds contain a good amount of monounsaturated fat and hunger-fighting proteins and leave you feeling full. The best way to include almonds in your diet is to add them to your daily bowl of smoothies, granola, or oats. That being said, you need to remember to consume almonds in moderation to contribute towards a balanced and healthy body.

Superfood 16: Quinoa

The moment you talk about "superfoods," the first thing that comes to my mind is quinoa. While the entire world is in a quest of sorts to search for the healthiest foods, you can't miss out on this ancient grain. Quinoa has slowly gained popularity in the past few years, making its way from the back shelves of the grocery store to being in the topmost supermarket aisles. This sweet and nutty flavored superfood is something all dieters swear by. This "mother of all grains" packs quite a punch with ample amounts of fiber, iron, potassium, magnesium, phosphorus, vitamin E, calcium, and a truckload of antioxidants. Quinoa is high in proteins, gluten-free, nutritious, and easy to digest.

One cup of quinoa consists of 6 g of fiber and 14 g of protein. This tiny grain has a mildly nutty flavor and a fluffy texture, which resembles couscous. Quinoa is packed with magnesium, which helps to relax your blood vessels and, as a result, alleviates the symptoms of migraines. It's also known to be effective in reducing the risk of type 2 diabetes, detoxifies your body, and promotes the formation of teeth and healthy bones. Its high manganese content offers plenty of antioxidants, thereby protecting the mitochondria from damage. Bodybuilders generally need to count the calories they consume with every meal, and eating quinoa for lunch can offer them the much-needed proteins for muscle repair and energy.

Superfood 17: Salmon

Sure, the classic hamburger or the popular hot dog makes for a tasty brunch, but they aren't really health friendly. If anything, they only end up adding some extra pounds, which are difficult to shake off. The very reason why people love junk food like pizzas or burgers is because they want something that excites their taste buds. If you are one of them, why not pile up on salmon? Sautéed or baked salmon, along with some herbs, can make a sumptuous spread.

Until some time ago, people started believing this myth that fat was some evil monster that could make you fat and be a probable cause of disease, but seriously, there's nothing to worry about consuming fatty fish like salmon. This fish is full of good fats, which protect your cardiovascular health, lower insulin resistance, prevent diabetes, and fight cancer.

Salmon is also high in omega-6 and omega-3 fatty acids, high-quality protein, minerals, and vitamins. You can buy salmon in the form of fillets or steaks, which can be canned, frozen, or smoked. Consuming fresh salmon on a regular basis can improve your skin, hair, and nails. If you are looking to develop some lean muscle, salmon could be your best bet as it's loaded with lean protein. You can add salmon to your curries, rice, noodles, pasta, and sandwiches, or simply grill it.

Superfood 18: Blueberries

My heart almost skips a beat when I spot a bunch of frozen blueberries lying on the kitchen table, especially during those hot summer afternoons. Blueberry juice makes for the perfect summer drink when you are in need of some hydration. Blueberries make a killer cocktail, too. These summer babies are an absolute favorite among kids. They are available in most grocery stores throughout the entire year but are slightly on the expensive side. Blueberries can be added to waffles, ice creams, smoothies, pies, and even breakfast oats.

The high level of anthocyanins, an antioxidant present in blueberries, helps in speeding up your metabolism, lowers blood pressure, and reduces the risk of coronary heart diseases. One cup of blueberries contains about 24% of the recommended vitamin C intake and 14% of recommended levels of fiber. They also prevent the growth of breast cancer cells in women's bodies.

Superfood 19: Pomegranate Seeds

While eating a pomegranate might mean a bit of work, dried pomegranate seeds are fuss-free. Pomegranates are a lovely fruit with juicy red jewels and a tiny little white seed in the middle. The fibrous seeds offer a variety of health benefits and make an ideal snack for people who like watching their weight. Pomegranate seeds contain a good number of antioxidants that help to fight against inflammation and aid in digestion. They are low in calories and high in potassium, vitamin C, fiber, folic acid, and iron. These little morsels are capable of boosting testosterone levels in men according to a study conducted in 2012. Some reports also started calling it the new Viagra. Half a cup of pomegranate seeds consists of about 4 g of fiber, 205 mg of potassium, and 14 micrograms of vitamin K.

Superfood 20: Oats

If there's one food that easily gets voted as the top favorite among all superfoods, it has to be the good ole "oats." That said, kids in particular often refer to oatmeal as tasteless and bland, but if you look closely, what's lurking in that bland bowl of porridge is some great p-oat-ential. Get it? Okay, no puns here. Packed with antioxidants, vitamins, nutrients, and minerals, oats make a high-fiber breakfast bowl that can provide you plenty of energy to roll throughout the day. It helps in lowering your cholesterol levels, enhances metabolism, improves digestion, and reduces the risk of heart disease.

Oatmeal can be consumed as a hot cereal or can be made into a delectable dessert (don't you love oatmeal Crème Brulee?). Oats are extremely popular among fitness lovers owing to their high protein and fiber content. One serving of oats contains as few as 50 calories, making it an ideal breakfast for weight watchers.

Conclusion

Let's not take pride in making statements like, "I am too busy to pay attention to my meals." I mean, what is so important that it takes precedence over your health? Let us all be responsible enough for our dietary needs, and let's inspire our kids to follow our path.

Making dietary changes could mean letting go of the most toxic foods that you have made a habit of eating on a daily basis. Of course, the journey isn't going to be easier unless you make a conscious decision to bring about a drastic change and then continue sticking to it. If you make healthy eating a lifestyle, you will no longer look at consuming superfoods as some form of punishment, but you will instead end up enjoying them.

Thank you, and remember to share how well these superfood tips work for you. You can do that by writing a review in your Amazon account under Your Orders.

Thank you,

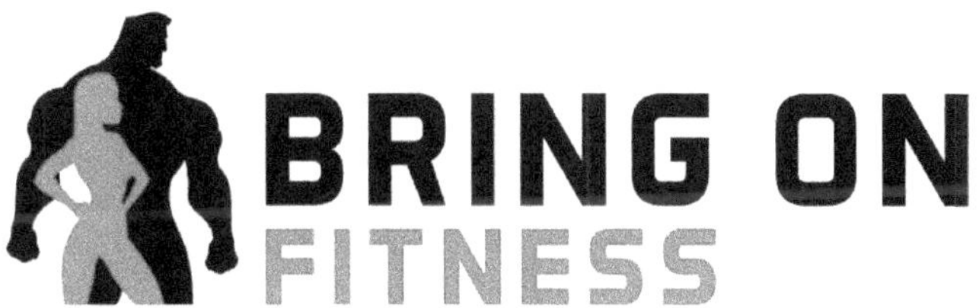

www.ingramcontent.com/pod-product-compliance
Lightning Source LLC
Chambersburg PA
CBHW070105260726
48658CB00002B/994